Gestational Diabetes Log Book

COPYRIGHT © 2017
ALL RIGHTS RESERVED.

ISBN-13: 978-1978435421
ISBN-10: 1978435428

D1468515

This Book Belong To:

Name _____

Address _____

_____

_____

Phone _____

Email _____

""

``

As a Reward: $

_____

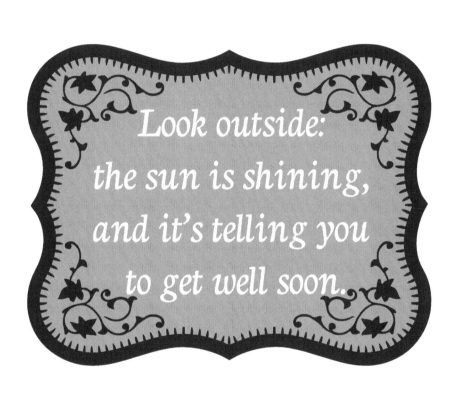

Look outside:
the sun is shining,
and it's telling you
to get well soon.

DAYS   **DATE**   **WEIGHT**

Sleep (Hrs) 🌙 1 2 3 4 5 6 7 8 _____
Water (Cup) 🥤🥤🥤🥤🥤🥤🥤🥤 _____

BREAKFAST	BEFORE	AFTER	CALORIES	CARBS (G)	ADDED SUGAR(G)	FIBER (G)	PROTEIN (G)	FAT (G)
TIME TOTAL:								
SNACK								
TIME TOTAL:								
LUNCH								
TIME TOTAL:								
SNACK								
TIME TOTAL:								

VITAMINS/MEDS/SUPPLEMENT/NOTES

DINNER	BEFORE	AFTER	CALORIES	CARBS (G)	ADDED SUGAR(G)	FIBER (G)	PROTEIN (G)	FAT (G)
TIME TOTAL:								
SNACK								
TIME TOTAL:								
GRAND TOTALS:								

PHYSICAL ACTIVITY

ACTIVITY	DURATION	INTENSITY	CAL/BURN

BLOOD SUGAR LOG

	BEFORE	AFTER	INSULIN

NOTES:

DAYS		DATE					WEIGHT		

SLEEP (HRS) 😴 1 2 3 4 5 6 7 8 _____
WATER (CUP) 🥤🥤🥤🥤🥤🥤🥤🥤 ____

BREAKFAST	BEFORE	AFTER	CALORIES	CARBS (G)	ADDED SUGAR(G)	FIBER (G)	PROTEIN (G)	FAT (G)
TIME TOTAL:								
SNACK								
TIME TOTAL:								
LUNCH								
TIME TOTAL:								
SNACK								
TIME TOTAL:								

VITAMINS/MEDS/SUPPLEMENT/NOTES

DINNER	BEFORE	AFTER	CALORIES	CARBS (G)	ADDED SUGAR(G)	FIBER (G)	PROTEIN (G)	FAT (G)
TIME TOTAL:								
SNACK								
TIME TOTAL:								
GRAND TOTALS:								

PHYSICAL ACTIVITY

ACTIVITY	DURATION	INTENSITY	CAL/BURN

BLOOD SUGAR LOG

	BEFORE	AFTER	INSULIN

NOTES:

DAYS   DATE   WEIGHT

Sleep (Hrs) 😴 1 2 3 4 5 6 7 8 ....
Water (Cup) 🥤🥤🥤🥤🥤🥤🥤🥤 ....

BREAKFAST	BEFORE	AFTER	Calories	Carbs (g)	Added Sugar(g)	Fiber (g)	Protein (g)	Fat (g)
Time Total:								
SNACK								
Time Total:								
LUNCH								
Time Total:								
SNACK								
Time Total:								

VITAMINS/MEDS/SUPPLEMENT/NOTES

DINNER	BEFORE	AFTER	CALORIES	CARBS (G)	ADDED SUGAR(G)	FIBER (G)	PROTEIN (G)	FAT (G)
TIME TOTAL:								
SNACK								
TIME TOTAL:								
GRAND TOTALS:								

PHYSICAL ACTIVITY

ACTIVITY	DURATION	INTENSITY	CAL/BURN

BLOOD SUGAR LOG

	BEFORE	AFTER	INSULIN

NOTES:

DAYS	DATE		WEIGHT

SLEEP (HRS) ☺ 1 2 3 4 5 6 7 8 ....
WATER (CUP) ⛾⛾⛾⛾⛾⛾⛾⛾⛾ ____

BREAKFAST	BEFORE	AFTER	CALORIES	CARBS (G)	ADDED SUGAR(G)	FIBER (G)	PROTEIN (G)	FAT (G)
TIME TOTAL:								
SNACK								
TIME TOTAL:								
LUNCH								
TIME TOTAL:								
SNACK								
TIME TOTAL:								

VITAMINS/MEDS/SUPPLEMENT/NOTES

DINNER	BEFORE	AFTER	CALORIES	CARBS (G)	ADDED SUGAR(G)	FIBER (G)	PROTEIN (G)	FAT (G)
⬛ME TOTAL:								
SNACK								
⬛ME TOTAL:								
GRAND TOTALS:								

PHYSICAL ACTIVITY

ACTIVITY	DURATION	INTENSITY	CAL/BURN

BLOOD SUGAR LOG

	BEFORE	AFTER	INSULIN

NOTES:

DAYS   DATE   WEIGHT

SLEEP (HRS) 😴 1 2 3 4 5 6 7 8 ......
WATER (CUP) 🥤🥤🥤🥤🥤🥤🥤🥤 ......

BREAKFAST	BEFORE	AFTER	CALORIES	CARBS (G)	ADDED SUGAR(G)	FIBER (G)	PROTEIN (G)	FAT (G)
TIME TOTAL:								
SNACK								
TIME TOTAL:								
LUNCH								
TIME TOTAL:								
SNACK								
TIME TOTAL:								

VITAMINS/MEDS/SUPPLEMENT/NOTES

DINNER	BEFORE	AFTER	CALORIES	CARBS (G)	ADDED SUGAR(G)	FIBER (G)	PROTEIN (G)	FAT (G)
TIME TOTAL:								
SNACK								
TIME TOTAL:								
GRAND TOTALS:								

PHYSICAL ACTIVITY

ACTIVITY	DURATION	INTENSITY	CAL/BURN

BLOOD SUGAR LOG

	BEFORE	AFTER	INSULIN

NOTES:

DAYS   DATE   WEIGHT

SLEEP (HRS) 🌙 1 2 3 4 5 6 7 8 ......
WATER (CUP) 🍵🍵🍵🍵🍵🍵🍵🍵 ____

BREAKFAST	BEFORE	AFTER	CALORIES	CARBS (G)	ADDED SUGAR(G)	FIBER (G)	PROTEIN (G)	FAT (G)
TIME TOTAL:								

SNACK								
TIME TOTAL:								

LUNCH								
TIME TOTAL:								

SNACK								
TIME TOTAL:								

VITAMINS/MEDS/SUPPLEMENT/NOTES

DINNER	BEFORE	AFTER	CALORIES	CARBS (G)	ADDED SUGAR(G)	FIBER (G)	PROTEIN (G)	FAT (G)
TIME TOTAL:								
SNACK								
TIME TOTAL:								
GRAND TOTALS:								

PHYSICAL ACTIVITY

ACTIVITY	DURATION	INTENSITY	CAL/BURN

BLOOD SUGAR LOG

	BEFORE	AFTER	INSULIN

NOTES:

DAYS　　　　**DATE**　　　　　　**WEIGHT**

SLEEP (HRS) 😴 1　2　3　4　5　6　7　8 _____
WATER (CUP) 🥤🥤🥤🥤🥤🥤🥤🥤 _____

BREAKFAST	BEFORE	AFTER	CALORIES	CARBS (G)	ADDED SUGAR(G)	FIBER (G)	PROTEIN (G)	FAT (G)
TIME　　　TOTAL:								
SNACK								
TIME　　　TOTAL:								
LUNCH								
TIME　　　TOTAL:								
SNACK								
TIME　　　TOTAL:								

VITAMINS/MEDS/SUPPLEMENT/NOTES

DINNER	BEFORE	AFTER	CALORIES	CARBS (G)	ADDED SUGAR(G)	FIBER (G)	PROTEIN (G)	FAT (G)
ME TOTAL:								

SNACK								
ME TOTAL:								
GRAND TOTALS:								

PHYSICAL ACTIVITY

ACTIVITY	DURATION	INTENSITY	CAL/BURN

BLOOD SUGAR LOG

	BEFORE	AFTER	INSULIN

NOTES:

DAYS DATE WEIGHT

SLEEP (HRS) 😴 1 2 3 4 5 6 7 8 _____
WATER (CUP) 🥤🥤🥤🥤🥤🥤🥤🥤 _____

BREAKFAST	BEFORE	AFTER	CALORIES	CARBS (G)	ADDED SUGAR(G)	FIBER (G)	PROTEIN (G)	FAT (G)
TIME TOTAL:								
SNACK								
TIME TOTAL:								
LUNCH								
TIME TOTAL:								
SNACK								
TIME TOTAL:								

VITAMINS/MEDS/SUPPLEMENT/NOTES

DINNER	BEFORE	AFTER	CALORIES	CARBS (G)	ADDED SUGAR(G)	FIBER (G)	PROTEIN (G)	FAT (G)
TIME TOTAL:								
SNACK								
TIME TOTAL:								
GRAND TOTALS:								

PHYSICAL ACTIVITY

ACTIVITY	DURATION	INTENSITY	CAL/BURN

BLOOD SUGAR LOG

	BEFORE	AFTER	INSULIN

NOTES:

DAYS   **DATE**   **WEIGHT**

SLEEP (HRS) 😴 1   2   3   4   5   6   7   8 ....
WATER (CUP) 🥤🥤🥤🥤🥤🥤🥤🥤 ....

BREAKFAST	BEFORE	AFTER	CALORIES	CARBS (G)	ADDED SUGAR(G)	FIBER (G)	PROTEIN (G)	FAT (G)
TIME TOTAL:								
SNACK								
TIME TOTAL:								
LUNCH								
TIME TOTAL:								
SNACK								
TIME TOTAL:								

VITAMINS/MEDS/SUPPLEMENT/NOTES

DINNER	BEFORE	AFTER	CALORIES	CARBS (G)	ADDED SUGAR(G)	FIBER (G)	PROTEIN (G)	FAT (G)
TIME TOTAL:								
SNACK								
TIME TOTAL:								
GRAND TOTALS:								

PHYSICAL ACTIVITY

ACTIVITY	DURATION	INTENSITY	CAL/BURN

BLOOD SUGAR LOG

	BEFORE	AFTER	INSULIN

NOTES:

DAYS   DATE   WEIGHT

SLEEP (HRS) 🌙 1 2 3 4 5 6 7 8 ....

WATER (CUP) ☕☕☕☕☕☕☕☕ ....

BREAKFAST	BEFORE	AFTER	CALORIES	CARBS (G)	ADDED SUGAR(G)	FIBER (G)	PROTEIN (G)	FAT (G)
TIME TOTAL:								
SNACK								
TIME TOTAL:								
LUNCH								
TIME TOTAL:								
SNACK								
TIME TOTAL:								

VITAMINS/MEDS/SUPPLEMENT/NOTES

DINNER	BEFORE	AFTER	CALORIES	CARBS (G)	ADDED SUGAR(G)	FIBER (G)	PROTEIN (G)	FAT (G)
TIME TOTAL:								
SNACK								
TIME TOTAL:								
GRAND TOTALS:								

PHYSICAL ACTIVITY

ACTIVITY	DURATION	INTENSITY	CAL/BURN

BLOOD SUGAR LOG

	BEFORE	AFTER	INSULIN

NOTES:

DAYS   DATE   WEIGHT

SLEEP (HRS) 1 2 3 4 5 6 7 8 ____
WATER (CUP) ◡◡◡◡◡◡◡◡ ____

BREAKFAST	BEFORE	AFTER	CALORIES	CARBS (G)	ADDED SUGAR(G)	FIBER (G)	PROTEIN (G)	FAT (G)
TIME TOTAL:								
SNACK								
TIME TOTAL:								
LUNCH								
TIME TOTAL:								
SNACK								
TIME TOTAL:								

VITAMINS/MEDS/SUPPLEMENT/NOTES

DINNER	BEFORE	AFTER	CALORIES	CARBS (G)	ADDED SUGAR(G)	FIBER (G)	PROTEIN (G)	FAT (G)
TIME TOTAL:								
SNACK								
TIME TOTAL:								
GRAND TOTALS:								

PHYSICAL ACTIVITY

ACTIVITY	DURATION	INTENSITY	CAL/BURN

BLOOD SUGAR LOG

	BEFORE	AFTER	INSULIN

NOTES:

DAYS   DATE   WEIGHT

SLEEP (HRS) 😴 1 2 3 4 5 6 7 8 ....
WATER (CUP) 🥤🥤🥤🥤🥤🥤🥤🥤🥤 ....

BREAKFAST	BEFORE	AFTER	CALORIES	CARBS (G)	ADDED SUGAR(G)	FIBER (G)	PROTEIN (G)	FAT (G)
TIME TOTAL:								
SNACK								
TIME TOTAL:								
LUNCH								
TIME TOTAL:								
SNACK								
TIME TOTAL:								

VITAMINS/MEDS/SUPPLEMENT/NOTES

DINNER	BEFORE	AFTER	CALORIES	CARBS (G)	ADDED SUGAR(G)	FIBER (G)	PROTEIN (G)	FAT (G)
TIME TOTAL:								
SNACK								
TIME TOTAL:								
GRAND TOTALS:								

PHYSICAL ACTIVITY

ACTIVITY	DURATION	INTENSITY	CAL/BURN

BLOOD SUGAR LOG

	BEFORE	AFTER	INSULIN

NOTES:

DAYS	DATE		WEIGHT	

SLEEP (HRS) 🌙 1 2 3 4 5 6 7 8 _____
WATER (CUP) 🍵🍵🍵🍵🍵🍵🍵🍵 _____

BREAKFAST	BEFORE	AFTER	CALORIES	CARBS (G)	ADDED SUGAR(G)	FIBER (G)	PROTEIN (G)	FAT (G)
TIME TOTAL:								
SNACK								
TIME TOTAL:								
LUNCH								
TIME TOTAL:								
SNACK								
TIME TOTAL:								

VITAMINS/MEDS/SUPPLEMENT/NOTES

DINNER	BEFORE	AFTER	CALORIES	CARBS (G)	ADDED SUGAR(G)	FIBER (G)	PROTEIN (G)	FAT (G)
TIME TOTAL:								
SNACK								
TIME TOTAL:								
GRAND TOTALS:								

PHYSICAL ACTIVITY

ACTIVITY	DURATION	INTENSITY	CAL/BURN

BLOOD SUGAR LOG

	BEFORE	AFTER	INSULIN

NOTES:

DAYS	DATE		WEIGHT

SLEEP (HRS) 😴 1 2 3 4 5 6 7 8 ____
WATER (CUP) 🥤🥤🥤🥤🥤🥤🥤🥤 ____

BREAKFAST	BEFORE	AFTER	CALORIES	CARBS (G)	ADDED SUGAR(G)	FIBER (G)	PROTEIN (G)	FAT (G)
TIME TOTAL:								
SNACK								
TIME TOTAL:								
LUNCH								
TIME TOTAL:								
SNACK								
TIME TOTAL:								

VITAMINS/MEDS/SUPPLEMENT/NOTES

DINNER	BEFORE	AFTER	CALORIES	CARBS (G)	ADDED SUGAR(G)	FIBER (G)	PROTEIN (G)	FAT (G)
TIME TOTAL:								
SNACK								
TIME TOTAL:								
GRAND TOTALS:								

PHYSICAL ACTIVITY

ACTIVITY	DURATION	INTENSITY	CAL/BURN

BLOOD SUGAR LOG

	BEFORE	AFTER	INSULIN

NOTES:

DAYS   **DATE**   **WEIGHT**

SLEEP (HRS) 😴 1 2 3 4 5 6 7 8 _____
WATER (CUP) 🥤🥤🥤🥤🥤🥤🥤🥤 _____

BREAKFAST	BEFORE	AFTER	CALORIES	CARBS (G)	ADDED SUGAR(G)	FIBER (G)	PROTEIN (G)	FAT (G)
TIME TOTAL:								
SNACK								
TIME TOTAL:								
LUNCH								
TIME TOTAL:								
SNACK								
TIME TOTAL:								

VITAMINS/MEDS/SUPPLEMENT/NOTES

DINNER	BEFORE	AFTER	CALORIES	CARBS (G)	ADDED SUGAR(G)	FIBER (G)	PROTEIN (G)	FAT (G)
TIME TOTAL:								
SNACK								
TIME TOTAL:								
GRAND TOTALS:								

PHYSICAL ACTIVITY

ACTIVITY	DURATION	INTENSITY	CAL/BURN

BLOOD SUGAR LOG

	BEFORE	AFTER	INSULIN

NOTES:

DAYS   DATE   WEIGHT

SLEEP (HRS) 😴 1 2 3 4 5 6 7 8 ....
WATER (CUP) 🥤🥤🥤🥤🥤🥤🥤🥤🥤 ....

BREAKFAST	BEFORE	AFTER	CALORIES	CARBS (G)	ADDED SUGAR(G)	FIBER (G)	PROTEIN (G)	FAT (G)
TIME TOTAL:								
SNACK								
TIME TOTAL:								
LUNCH								
TIME TOTAL:								
SNACK								
TIME TOTAL:								

VITAMINS/MEDS/SUPPLEMENT/NOTES

DINNER	BEFORE	AFTER	CALORIES	CARBS (G)	ADDED SUGAR(G)	FIBER (G)	PROTEIN (G)	FAT (G)
TIME TOTAL:								
SNACK								
TIME TOTAL:								
GRAND TOTALS:								

PHYSICAL ACTIVITY

ACTIVITY	DURATION	INTENSITY	CAL/BURN

BLOOD SUGAR LOG

	BEFORE	AFTER	INSULIN

NOTES:

DAYS   DATE   WEIGHT

SLEEP (HRS) 😴 1 2 3 4 5 6 7 8 ....
WATER (CUP) 🥤🥤🥤🥤🥤🥤🥤🥤 ....

BREAKFAST	BEFORE	AFTER	CALORIES	CARBS (G)	ADDED SUGAR(G)	FIBER (G)	PROTEIN (G)	FAT (G)
TIME TOTAL:								
SNACK								
TIME TOTAL:								
LUNCH								
TIME TOTAL:								
SNACK								
TIME TOTAL:								

VITAMINS/MEDS/SUPPLEMENT/NOTES

DINNER	BEFORE	AFTER	CALORIES	CARBS (G)	ADDED SUGAR(G)	FIBER (G)	PROTEIN (G)	FAT (G)
TIME TOTAL:								
SNACK								
TIME TOTAL:								
GRAND TOTALS:								

PHYSICAL ACTIVITY

ACTIVITY	DURATION	INTENSITY	CAL/BURN

BLOOD SUGAR LOG

	BEFORE	AFTER	INSULIN

NOTES:

DAYS   **DATE**   **WEIGHT**

SLEEP (HRS) 😴 1   2   3   4   5   6   7   8 _____
WATER (CUP) 🥤🥤🥤🥤🥤🥤🥤🥤 ____

BREAKFAST	BEFORE	AFTER	CALORIES	CARBS (G)	ADDED SUGAR(G)	FIBER (G)	PROTEIN (G)	FAT (G)
TIME TOTAL:								
SNACK								
TIME TOTAL:								
LUNCH								
TIME TOTAL:								
SNACK								
TIME TOTAL:								

VITAMINS/MEDS/SUPPLEMENT/NOTES

DINNER	BEFORE	AFTER	CALORIES	CARBS (G)	ADDED SUGAR(G)	FIBER (G)	PROTEIN (G)	FAT (G)
TIME TOTAL:								
SNACK								
TIME TOTAL:								
GRAND TOTALS:								

PHYSICAL ACTIVITY

ACTIVITY	DURATION	INTENSITY	CAL/BURN

BLOOD SUGAR LOG

	BEFORE	AFTER	INSULIN

NOTES:

DAYS   **DATE**   **WEIGHT**

SLEEP (HRS) ☺ 1 2 3 4 5 6 7 8 ....
WATER (CUP) ☕☕☕☕☕☕☕☕ ....

BREAKFAST	BEFORE	AFTER	CALORIES	CARBS (G)	ADDED SUGAR(G)	FIBER (G)	PROTEIN (G)	FAT (G)
TIME TOTAL:								
SNACK								
TIME TOTAL:								
LUNCH								
TIME TOTAL:								
SNACK								
TIME TOTAL:								

VITAMINS/MEDS/SUPPLEMENT/NOTES

DINNER	BEFORE	AFTER	CALORIES	CARBS (G)	ADDED SUGAR(G)	FIBER (G)	PROTEIN (G)	FAT (G)
TIME TOTAL:								
SNACK								
TIME TOTAL:								
GRAND TOTALS:								

PHYSICAL ACTIVITY

ACTIVITY	DURATION	INTENSITY	CAL/BURN

BLOOD SUGAR LOG

	BEFORE	AFTER	INSULIN

NOTES:

DAYS   DATE   WEIGHT

SLEEP (HRS) 🌙 1 2 3 4 5 6 7 8 ....
WATER (CUP) 🍵🍵🍵🍵🍵🍵🍵🍵 ....

BREAKFAST	BEFORE	AFTER	CALORIES	CARBS (G)	ADDED SUGAR(G)	FIBER (G)	PROTEIN (G)	FAT (G)
TIME TOTAL:								
SNACK								
TIME TOTAL:								
LUNCH								
TIME TOTAL:								
SNACK								
TIME TOTAL:								

VITAMINS/MEDS/SUPPLEMENT/NOTES

DINNER	BEFORE	AFTER	CALORIES	CARBS (G)	ADDED SUGAR(G)	FIBER (G)	PROTEIN (G)	FAT (G)
ME TOTAL:								
SNACK								
ME TOTAL:								
GRAND TOTALS:								

PHYSICAL ACTIVITY

ACTIVITY	DURATION	INTENSITY	CAL/BURN

BLOOD SUGAR LOG

	BEFORE	AFTER	INSULIN

NOTES:

DAYS   DATE   WEIGHT

SLEEP (HRS) 🌙 1 2 3 4 5 6 7 8 ....
WATER (CUP) ⊌ ⊌ ⊌ ⊌ ⊌ ⊌ ⊌ ⊌ ⊌ ....

BREAKFAST	BEFORE	AFTER	CALORIES	CARBS (G)	ADDED SUGAR(G)	FIBER (G)	PROTEIN (G)	FAT (G)
TIME TOTAL:								
SNACK								
TIME TOTAL:								
LUNCH								
TIME TOTAL:								
SNACK								
TIME TOTAL:								

VITAMINS/MEDS/SUPPLEMENT/NOTES

DINNER	BEFORE	AFTER	CALORIES	CARBS (G)	ADDED SUGAR(G)	FIBER (G)	PROTEIN (G)	FAT (G)
TIME TOTAL:								
SNACK								
TIME TOTAL:								
GRAND TOTALS:								

PHYSICAL ACTIVITY

ACTIVITY	DURATION	INTENSITY	CAL/BURN

BLOOD SUGAR LOG

	BEFORE	AFTER	INSULIN

NOTES:

DAYS   DATE   WEIGHT

SLEEP (HRS) 😴 1   2   3   4   5   6   7   8 ....

WATER (CUP) 🥤🥤🥤🥤🥤🥤🥤🥤 ....

BREAKFAST	BEFORE	AFTER	CALORIES	CARBS (G)	ADDED SUGAR(G)	FIBER (G)	PROTEIN (G)	FAT (G)
TIME TOTAL:								
SNACK								
TIME TOTAL:								
LUNCH								
TIME TOTAL:								
SNACK								
TIME TOTAL:								

VITAMINS/MEDS/SUPPLEMENT/NOTES

DINNER	BEFORE	AFTER	CALORIES	CARBS (G)	ADDED SUGAR(G)	FIBER (G)	PROTEIN (G)	FAT (G)
TIME TOTAL:								
SNACK								
TIME TOTAL:								
GRAND TOTALS:								

PHYSICAL ACTIVITY

ACTIVITY	DURATION	INTENSITY	CAL/BURN

BLOOD SUGAR LOG

	BEFORE	AFTER	INSULIN

NOTES:

DAYS	DATE		WEIGHT

SLEEP (HRS) 😴 1 2 3 4 5 6 7 8 _____
WATER (CUP) 🥛🥛🥛🥛🥛🥛🥛🥛 _____

BREAKFAST	BEFORE	AFTER	CALORIES	CARBS (G)	ADDED SUGAR(G)	FIBER (G)	PROTEIN (G)	FAT (G)
TIME TOTAL:								
SNACK								
TIME TOTAL:								
LUNCH								
TIME TOTAL:								
SNACK								
TIME TOTAL:								

VITAMINS/MEDS/SUPPLEMENT/NOTES

DINNER	BEFORE	AFTER	CALORIES	CARBS (G)	ADDED SUGAR(G)	FIBER (G)	PROTEIN (G)	FAT (G)
TIME TOTAL:								
SNACK								
TIME TOTAL:								
GRAND TOTALS:								

PHYSICAL ACTIVITY

ACTIVITY	DURATION	INTENSITY	CAL/BURN

BLOOD SUGAR LOG

	BEFORE	AFTER	INSULIN

NOTES:

DAYS	DATE		WEIGHT	

SLEEP (HRS) 🌙 1 2 3 4 5 6 7 8 _____
WATER (CUP) 🥤🥤🥤🥤🥤🥤🥤🥤 _____

BREAKFAST	BEFORE	AFTER	CALORIES	CARBS (G)	ADDED SUGAR(G)	FIBER (G)	PROTEIN (G)	FAT (G)
TIME TOTAL:								
SNACK								
TIME TOTAL:								
LUNCH								
TIME TOTAL:								
SNACK								
TIME TOTAL:								

VITAMINS/MEDS/SUPPLEMENT/NOTES

DINNER	BEFORE	AFTER	CALORIES	CARBS (G)	ADDED SUGAR(G)	FIBER (G)	PROTEIN (G)	FAT (G)
TIME TOTAL:								
SNACK								
TIME TOTAL:								
GRAND TOTALS:								

PHYSICAL ACTIVITY

ACTIVITY	DURATION	INTENSITY	CAL/BURN

BLOOD SUGAR LOG

	BEFORE	AFTER	INSULIN

NOTES:

DAYS   DATE   WEIGHT

SLEEP (HRS) 🌙 1 2 3 4 5 6 7 8 ....
WATER (CUP) 🥤🥤🥤🥤🥤🥤🥤🥤 ....

BREAKFAST	BEFORE	AFTER	CALORIES	CARBS (G)	ADDED SUGAR(G)	FIBER (G)	PROTEIN (G)	FAT (G)
TIME TOTAL:								
SNACK								
TIME TOTAL:								
LUNCH								
TIME TOTAL:								
SNACK								
TIME TOTAL:								

VITAMINS/MEDS/SUPPLEMENT/NOTES

DINNER	BEFORE	AFTER	CALORIES	CARBS (G)	ADDED SUGAR(G)	FIBER (G)	PROTEIN (G)	FAT (G)
TIME TOTAL:								
SNACK								
TIME TOTAL:								
GRAND TOTALS:								

PHYSICAL ACTIVITY

ACTIVITY	DURATION	INTENSITY	CAL/BURN

BLOOD SUGAR LOG

	BEFORE	AFTER	INSULIN

NOTES:

DAYS   DATE   WEIGHT

SLEEP (HRS) 😴 1 2 3 4 5 6 7 8 ____
WATER (CUP) 🥛🥛🥛🥛🥛🥛🥛🥛 ____

BREAKFAST	BEFORE	AFTER	CALORIES	CARBS (G)	ADDED SUGAR(G)	FIBER (G)	PROTEIN (G)	FAT (G)
TIME TOTAL:								

SNACK								
TIME TOTAL:								

LUNCH								
TIME TOTAL:								

SNACK								
TIME TOTAL:								

VITAMINS/MEDS/SUPPLEMENT/NOTES

DINNER	BEFORE	AFTER	CALORIES	CARBS (G)	ADDED SUGAR(G)	FIBER (G)	PROTEIN (G)	FAT (G)
TIME TOTAL:								
SNACK								
TIME TOTAL:								
GRAND TOTALS:								

PHYSICAL ACTIVITY

ACTIVITY	DURATION	INTENSITY	CAL/BURN

BLOOD SUGAR LOG

	BEFORE	AFTER	INSULIN

NOTES:

DAYS　　　**DATE**　　　　　　　**WEIGHT**

SLEEP (HRS) 🌙 1　2　3　4　5　6　7　8 _____
WATER (CUP) 🥛🥛🥛🥛🥛🥛🥛🥛 _____

BREAKFAST	BEFORE	AFTER	CALORIES	CARBS (G)	ADDED SUGAR(G)	FIBER (G)	PROTEIN (G)	FAT (G)
TIME　　　TOTAL:								
SNACK								
TIME　　　TOTAL:								
LUNCH								
TIME　　　TOTAL:								
SNACK								
TIME　　　TOTAL:								

VITAMINS/MEDS/SUPPLEMENT/NOTES

DINNER	BEFORE	AFTER	CALORIES	CARBS (G)	ADDED SUGAR(G)	FIBER (G)	PROTEIN (G)	FAT (G)
TIME TOTAL:								
SNACK								
TIME TOTAL:								
GRAND TOTALS:								

PHYSICAL ACTIVITY

ACTIVITY	DURATION	INTENSITY	CAL/BURN

BLOOD SUGAR LOG

	BEFORE	AFTER	INSULIN

NOTES:

DAYS	DATE		WEIGHT	

SLEEP (HRS) 🌙 1 2 3 4 5 6 7 8 _____
WATER (CUP) 🥤🥤🥤🥤🥤🥤🥤🥤 ____

BREAKFAST	BEFORE	AFTER	CALORIES	CARBS (G)	ADDED SUGAR(G)	FIBER (G)	PROTEIN (G)	FAT (G)
TIME TOTAL:								
SNACK								
TIME TOTAL:								
LUNCH								
TIME TOTAL:								
SNACK								
TIME TOTAL:								

VITAMINS/MEDS/SUPPLEMENT/NOTES

DINNER	BEFORE	AFTER	CALORIES	CARBS (G)	ADDED SUGAR(G)	FIBER (G)	PROTEIN (G)	FAT (G)
TIME TOTAL:								
SNACK								
TIME TOTAL:								
GRAND TOTALS:								

PHYSICAL ACTIVITY

ACTIVITY	DURATION	INTENSITY	CAL/BURN

BLOOD SUGAR LOG

	BEFORE	AFTER	INSULIN

NOTES:

DAYS   DATE   WEIGHT

SLEEP (HRS) 🕐 1 2 3 4 5 6 7 8 ....
WATER (CUP) ⊂⊃ ⊂⊃ ⊂⊃ ⊂⊃ ⊂⊃ ⊂⊃ ⊂⊃ ⊂⊃ ____

BREAKFAST	BEFORE	AFTER	CALORIES	CARBS (G)	ADDED SUGAR(G)	FIBER (G)	PROTEIN (G)	FAT (G)
TIME TOTAL:								
SNACK								
TIME TOTAL:								
LUNCH								
TIME TOTAL:								
SNACK								
TIME TOTAL:								

VITAMINS/MEDS/SUPPLEMENT/NOTES

DINNER	BEFORE	AFTER	CALORIES	CARBS (G)	ADDED SUGAR(G)	FIBER (G)	PROTEIN (G)	FAT (G)
TIME TOTAL:								
SNACK								
TIME TOTAL:								
GRAND TOTALS:								

PHYSICAL ACTIVITY

ACTIVITY	DURATION	INTENSITY	CAL/BURN

BLOOD SUGAR LOG

	BEFORE	AFTER	INSULIN

NOTES:

DAYS		DATE			WEIGHT		

SLEEP (HRS) 😴 1 2 3 4 5 6 7 8 ....
WATER (CUP) 🥤🥤🥤🥤🥤🥤🥤🥤 ___

BREAKFAST	BEFORE	AFTER	CALORIES	CARBS (G)	ADDED SUGAR(G)	FIBER (G)	PROTEIN (G)	FAT (G)
TIME TOTAL:								
SNACK								
TIME TOTAL:								
LUNCH								
TIME TOTAL:								
SNACK								
TIME TOTAL:								

VITAMINS/MEDS/SUPPLEMENT/NOTES

DINNER	BEFORE	AFTER	CALORIES	CARBS (G)	ADDED SUGAR(G)	FIBER (G)	PROTEIN (G)	FAT (G)
TIME TOTAL:								
SNACK								
TIME TOTAL:								
GRAND TOTALS:								

PHYSICAL ACTIVITY

ACTIVITY	DURATION	INTENSITY	CAL/BURN

BLOOD SUGAR LOG

	BEFORE	AFTER	INSULIN

NOTES:

DAYS   DATE   WEIGHT

SLEEP (HRS) 🛌 1 2 3 4 5 6 7 8 _____
WATER (CUP) 🥤🥤🥤🥤🥤🥤🥤🥤 ____

BREAKFAST	BEFORE	AFTER	CALORIES	CARBS (G)	ADDED SUGAR(G)	FIBER (G)	PROTEIN (G)	FAT (G)
TIME TOTAL:								
SNACK								
TIME TOTAL:								
LUNCH								
TIME TOTAL:								
SNACK								
TIME TOTAL:								

VITAMINS/MEDS/SUPPLEMENT/NOTES

DINNER	Before	After	Calories	Carbs (G)	Added Sugar(G)	Fiber (G)	Protein (G)	Fat (G)
ME TOTAL:								
SNACK								
ME TOTAL:								
GRAND TOTALS:								

PHYSICAL ACTIVITY

ACTIVITY	DURATION	INTENSITY	CAL/BURN

BLOOD SUGAR LOG

	BEFORE	AFTER	INSULIN

NOTES:

DAYS   DATE   WEIGHT

SLEEP (HRS) 🕐 1 2 3 4 5 6 7 8 _____
WATER (CUP) ▭▭▭▭▭▭▭▭ _____

BREAKFAST	BEFORE	AFTER	CALORIES	CARBS (G)	ADDED SUGAR(G)	FIBER (G)	PROTEIN (G)	FAT (G
TIME TOTAL:								
SNACK								
TIME TOTAL:								
LUNCH								
TIME TOTAL:								
SNACK								
TIME TOTAL:								

VITAMINS/MEDS/SUPPLEMENT/NOTES

DINNER	BEFORE	AFTER	CALORIES	CARBS (G)	ADDED SUGAR(G)	FIBER (G)	PROTEIN (G)	FAT (G)
TIME TOTAL:								
SNACK								
TIME TOTAL:								
GRAND TOTALS:								

PHYSICAL ACTIVITY

ACTIVITY	DURATION	INTENSITY	CAL/BURN

BLOOD SUGAR LOG

	BEFORE	AFTER	INSULIN

NOTES:

DAYS	DATE		WEIGHT	

SLEEP (HRS) 🛌 1 2 3 4 5 6 7 8 _____
WATER (CUP) 🥛🥛🥛🥛🥛🥛🥛🥛 ____

BREAKFAST	BEFORE	AFTER	CALORIES	CARBS (G)	ADDED SUGAR(G)	FIBER (G)	PROTEIN (G)	FAT (G)
TIME TOTAL:								
SNACK								
TIME TOTAL:								
LUNCH								
TIME TOTAL:								
SNACK								
TIME TOTAL:								

VITAMINS/MEDS/SUPPLEMENT/NOTES

DINNER	BEFORE	AFTER	CALORIES	CARBS (G)	ADDED SUGAR(G)	FIBER (G)	PROTEIN (G)	FAT (G)
TIME TOTAL:								
SNACK								
TIME TOTAL:								
GRAND TOTALS:								

PHYSICAL ACTIVITY

ACTIVITY	DURATION	INTENSITY	CAL/BURN

BLOOD SUGAR LOG

	BEFORE	AFTER	INSULIN

NOTES:

DAYS | **DATE** | **WEIGHT**

SLEEP (HRS) 😴 1 2 3 4 5 6 7 8 ....
WATER (CUP) 🥛🥛🥛🥛🥛🥛🥛🥛 ....

BREAKFAST	BEFORE	AFTER	CALORIES	CARBS (G)	ADDED SUGAR(G)	FIBER (G)	PROTEIN (G)	FAT (G)
TIME TOTAL:								
SNACK								
TIME TOTAL:								
LUNCH								
TIME TOTAL:								
SNACK								
TIME TOTAL:								

VITAMINS/MEDS/SUPPLEMENT/NOTES

DINNER	BEFORE	AFTER	CALORIES	CARBS (G)	ADDED SUGAR(G)	FIBER (G)	PROTEIN (G)	FAT (G)
TIME TOTAL:								
SNACK								
TIME TOTAL:								
GRAND TOTALS:								

PHYSICAL ACTIVITY

ACTIVITY	DURATION	INTENSITY	CAL/BURN

BLOOD SUGAR LOG

	BEFORE	AFTER	INSULIN

NOTES:

DAYS   **DATE**   **WEIGHT**

SLEEP (HRS) 🌙 1 2 3 4 5 6 7 8 ....
WATER (CUP) ◖◖◖◖◖◖◖◖ ____

BREAKFAST	BEFORE	AFTER	CALORIES	CARBS (G)	ADDED SUGAR(G)	FIBER (G)	PROTEIN (G)	FAT (G)
TIME _____ TOTAL:								
SNACK								
TIME _____ TOTAL:								
LUNCH								
TIME _____ TOTAL:								
SNACK								
TIME _____ TOTAL:								

VITAMINS/MEDS/SUPPLEMENT/NOTES

DINNER	BEFORE	AFTER	CALORIES	CARBS (G)	ADDED SUGAR(G)	FIBER (G)	PROTEIN (G)	FAT (G)
TIME TOTAL:								
SNACK								
TIME TOTAL:								
GRAND TOTALS:								

PHYSICAL ACTIVITY

ACTIVITY	DURATION	INTENSITY	CAL/BURN

BLOOD SUGAR LOG

	BEFORE	AFTER	INSULIN

NOTES:

DAYS   DATE   WEIGHT

SLEEP (HRS) 🌙 1 2 3 4 5 6 7 8 _____
WATER (CUP) ⊂⊃⊂⊃⊂⊃⊂⊃⊂⊃⊂⊃⊂⊃⊂⊃ _____

BREAKFAST	BEFORE	AFTER	CALORIES	CARBS (G)	ADDED SUGAR(G)	FIBER (G)	PROTEIN (G)	FAT (G)
TIME TOTAL:								
SNACK								
TIME TOTAL:								
LUNCH								
TIME TOTAL:								
SNACK								
TIME TOTAL:								

VITAMINS/MEDS/SUPPLEMENT/NOTES

DINNER	BEFORE	AFTER	CALORIES	CARBS (G)	ADDED SUGAR(G)	FIBER (G)	PROTEIN (G)	FAT (G)
TIME TOTAL:								
SNACK								
TIME TOTAL:								
GRAND TOTALS:								

PHYSICAL ACTIVITY

ACTIVITY	DURATION	INTENSITY	CAL/BURN

BLOOD SUGAR LOG

	BEFORE	AFTER	INSULIN

NOTES:

DAYS   **DATE**   **WEIGHT**

SLEEP (HRS) 🌙 1 2 3 4 5 6 7 8 ____
WATER (CUP) 🍵🍵🍵🍵🍵🍵🍵🍵 ____

BREAKFAST	BEFORE	AFTER	CALORIES	CARBS (G)	ADDED SUGAR(G)	FIBER (G)	PROTEIN (G)	FAT (G)
TIME TOTAL:								
SNACK								
TIME TOTAL:								
LUNCH								
TIME TOTAL:								
SNACK								
TIME TOTAL:								

VITAMINS/MEDS/SUPPLEMENT/NOTES

DINNER	BEFORE	AFTER	CALORIES	CARBS (G)	ADDED SUGAR(G)	FIBER (G)	PROTEIN (G)	FAT (G)
TIME TOTAL:								
SNACK								
TIME TOTAL:								
GRAND TOTALS:								

PHYSICAL ACTIVITY

ACTIVITY	DURATION	INTENSITY	CAL/BURN

BLOOD SUGAR LOG

	BEFORE	AFTER	INSULIN

NOTES:

DAYS   DATE   WEIGHT

SLEEP (HRS) 🕑 1 2 3 4 5 6 7 8 ____
WATER (CUP) ☕☕☕☕☕☕☕☕ ____

BREAKFAST	BEFORE	AFTER	CALORIES	CARBS (G)	ADDED SUGAR(G)	FIBER (G)	PROTEIN (G)	FAT (G)
TIME TOTAL:								
SNACK								
TIME TOTAL:								
LUNCH								
TIME TOTAL:								
SNACK								
TIME TOTAL:								

VITAMINS/MEDS/SUPPLEMENT/NOTES

DINNER	BEFORE	AFTER	CALORIES	CARBS (G)	ADDED SUGAR(G)	FIBER (G)	PROTEIN (G)	FAT (G)
TIME TOTAL:								
SNACK								
TIME TOTAL:								
GRAND TOTALS:								

PHYSICAL ACTIVITY

ACTIVITY	DURATION	INTENSITY	CAL/BURN

BLOOD SUGAR LOG

	BEFORE	AFTER	INSULIN

NOTES:

DAYS		DATE					WEIGHT		

SLEEP (HRS) 🌙 1 2 3 4 5 6 7 8 _____
WATER (CUP) 🥛🥛🥛🥛🥛🥛🥛🥛 _____

BREAKFAST	BEFORE	AFTER	CALORIES	CARBS (G)	ADDED SUGAR(G)	FIBER (G)	PROTEIN (G)	FAT (G)
TIME TOTAL:								
SNACK								
TIME TOTAL:								
LUNCH								
TIME TOTAL:								
SNACK								
TIME TOTAL:								

VITAMINS/MEDS/SUPPLEMENT/NOTES

DINNER	BEFORE	AFTER	CALORIES	CARBS (G)	ADDED SUGAR(G)	FIBER (G)	PROTEIN (G)	FAT (G)
TIME TOTAL:								
SNACK								
TIME TOTAL:								
GRAND TOTALS:								

PHYSICAL ACTIVITY

ACTIVITY	DURATION	INTENSITY	CAL/BURN

BLOOD SUGAR LOG

	BEFORE	AFTER	INSULIN

NOTES:

DAYS	DATE		WEIGHT	

SLEEP (HRS) 😴 1 2 3 4 5 6 7 8 _____
WATER (CUP) 🥤🥤🥤🥤🥤🥤🥤🥤 _____

BREAKFAST	BEFORE	AFTER	CALORIES	CARBS (G)	ADDED SUGAR(G)	FIBER (G)	PROTEIN (G)	FAT (G)
TIME TOTAL:								
SNACK								
TIME TOTAL:								
LUNCH								
TIME TOTAL:								
SNACK								
TIME TOTAL:								

VITAMINS/MEDS/SUPPLEMENT/NOTES

DINNER	BEFORE	AFTER	CALORIES	CARBS (G)	ADDED SUGAR(G)	FIBER (G)	PROTEIN (G)	FAT (G)
ME TOTAL:								
SNACK								
ME TOTAL:								
GRAND TOTALS:								

PHYSICAL ACTIVITY

ACTIVITY	DURATION	INTENSITY	CAL/BURN

BLOOD SUGAR LOG

	BEFORE	AFTER	INSULIN

NOTES:

DAYS [ ]   DATE [ ]   WEIGHT [ ]

SLEEP (HRS) 🕐 1 2 3 4 5 6 7 8 ....
WATER (CUP) 🥤🥤🥤🥤🥤🥤🥤🥤 ....

BREAKFAST	BEFORE	AFTER	CALORIES	CARBS (G)	ADDED SUGAR(G)	FIBER (G)	PROTEIN (G)	FAT (G)
TIME _____ TOTAL:								
SNACK								
TIME _____ TOTAL:								
LUNCH								
TIME _____ TOTAL:								
SNACK								
TIME _____ TOTAL:								

VITAMINS/MEDS/SUPPLEMENT/NOTES

DINNER	BEFORE	AFTER	CALORIES	CARBS (G)	ADDED SUGAR(G)	FIBER (G)	PROTEIN (G)	FAT (G)
TIME TOTAL:								
SNACK								
TIME TOTAL:								
GRAND TOTALS:								

PHYSICAL ACTIVITY

ACTIVITY	DURATION	INTENSITY	CAL/BURN

BLOOD SUGAR LOG

	BEFORE	AFTER	INSULIN

NOTES:

DAYS		DATE		WEIGHT	

SLEEP (HRS) 🌙 1 2 3 4 5 6 7 8 _____
WATER (CUP) 🥤🥤🥤🥤🥤🥤🥤🥤 _____

BREAKFAST	BEFORE	AFTER	CALORIES	CARBS (G)	ADDED SUGAR(G)	FIBER (G)	PROTEIN (G)	FAT (G)
TIME TOTAL:								
SNACK								
TIME TOTAL:								
LUNCH								
TIME TOTAL:								
SNACK								
TIME TOTAL:								

VITAMINS/MEDS/SUPPLEMENT/NOTES

DINNER	BEFORE	AFTER	CALORIES	CARBS (G)	ADDED SUGAR(G)	FIBER (G)	PROTEIN (G)	FAT (G)
ME TOTAL:								
SNACK								
ME TOTAL:								
GRAND TOTALS:								

PHYSICAL ACTIVITY

ACTIVITY	DURATION	INTENSITY	CAL/BURN

BLOOD SUGAR LOG

	BEFORE	AFTER	INSULIN

NOTES:

DAYS   DATE   WEIGHT

SLEEP (HRS) 🌙 1 2 3 4 5 6 7 8 _____
WATER (CUP) 🥤🥤🥤🥤🥤🥤🥤🥤 ____

BREAKFAST	BEFORE	AFTER	CALORIES	CARBS (G)	ADDED SUGAR(G)	FIBER (G)	PROTEIN (G)	FAT (G)
TIME TOTAL:								
SNACK								
TIME TOTAL:								
LUNCH								
TIME TOTAL:								
SNACK								
TIME TOTAL:								

VITAMINS/MEDS/SUPPLEMENT/NOTES

DINNER	BEFORE	AFTER	CALORIES	CARBS (G)	ADDED SUGAR(G)	FIBER (G)	PROTEIN (G)	FAT (G)
TIME TOTAL:								
SNACK								
TIME TOTAL:								
GRAND TOTALS:								

PHYSICAL ACTIVITY

ACTIVITY	DURATION	INTENSITY	CAL/BURN

BLOOD SUGAR LOG

	BEFORE	AFTER	INSULIN

NOTES:

DAYS   **DATE**   **WEIGHT**

SLEEP (HRS) 🔆 1 2 3 4 5 6 7 8 ___
WATER (CUP) ▭▭▭▭▭▭▭▭ ___

BREAKFAST	BEFORE	AFTER	CALORIES	CARBS (G)	ADDED SUGAR(G)	FIBER (G)	PROTEIN (G)	FAT (G)
TIME TOTAL:								
SNACK								
TIME TOTAL:								
LUNCH								
TIME TOTAL:								
SNACK								
TIME TOTAL:								

VITAMINS/MEDS/SUPPLEMENT/NOTES

DINNER	BEFORE	AFTER	CALORIES	CARBS (G)	ADDED SUGAR(G)	FIBER (G)	PROTEIN (G)	FAT (G)
TIME TOTAL:								
SNACK								
TIME TOTAL:								
GRAND TOTALS:								

PHYSICAL ACTIVITY

ACTIVITY	DURATION	INTENSITY	CAL/BURN

BLOOD SUGAR LOG

	BEFORE	AFTER	INSULIN

NOTES:

DAYS   **DATE**   **WEIGHT**

SLEEP (HRS) 1 2 3 4 5 6 7 8 ......
WATER (CUP) ◠ ◠ ◠ ◠ ◠ ◠ ◠ ◠ ◠ ____

BREAKFAST	BEFORE	AFTER	CALORIES	CARBS (G)	ADDED SUGAR(G)	FIBER (G)	PROTEIN (G)	FAT (G)
TIME TOTAL:								
SNACK								
TIME TOTAL:								
LUNCH								
TIME TOTAL:								
SNACK								
TIME TOTAL:								

VITAMINS/MEDS/SUPPLEMENT/NOTES

DINNER	BEFORE	AFTER	CALORIES	CARBS (G)	ADDED SUGAR(G)	FIBER (G)	PROTEIN (G)	FAT (G)
TIME TOTAL:								
SNACK								
TIME TOTAL:								
GRAND TOTALS:								

PHYSICAL ACTIVITY

ACTIVITY	DURATION	INTENSITY	CAL/BURN

BLOOD SUGAR LOG

	BEFORE	AFTER	INSULIN

NOTES:

DAYS	DATE		WEIGHT	

SLEEP (HRS) 🕐 1 2 3 4 5 6 7 8 ____
WATER (CUP) 🥤🥤🥤🥤🥤🥤🥤🥤🥤 ____

BREAKFAST	BEFORE	AFTER	CALORIES	CARBS (G)	ADDED SUGAR(G)	FIBER (G)	PROTEIN (G)	FAT (G)
TIME TOTAL:								
SNACK								
TIME TOTAL:								
LUNCH								
TIME TOTAL:								
SNACK								
TIME TOTAL:								

VITAMINS/MEDS/SUPPLEMENT/NOTES

DINNER	BEFORE	AFTER	CALORIES	CARBS (G)	ADDED SUGAR(G)	FIBER (G)	PROTEIN (G)	FAT (G)
TIME TOTAL:								
SNACK								
TIME TOTAL:								
GRAND TOTALS:								

PHYSICAL ACTIVITY

ACTIVITY	DURATION	INTENSITY	CAL/BURN

BLOOD SUGAR LOG

	BEFORE	AFTER	INSULIN

NOTES:

DAYS   DATE   WEIGHT

SLEEP (HRS) 🌙 1 2 3 4 5 6 7 8 ____
WATER (CUP) ⊂⊃⊂⊃⊂⊃⊂⊃⊂⊃⊂⊃⊂⊃⊂⊃ ____

BREAKFAST	BEFORE	AFTER	CALORIES	CARBS (G)	ADDED SUGAR(G)	FIBER (G)	PROTEIN (G)	FAT (G)
TIME TOTAL:								

SNACK								
TIME TOTAL:								

LUNCH								
TIME TOTAL:								

SNACK								
TIME TOTAL:								

VITAMINS/MEDS/SUPPLEMENT/NOTES

DINNER	BEFORE	AFTER	CALORIES	CARBS (G)	ADDED SUGAR(G)	FIBER (G)	PROTEIN (G)	FAT (G)
TIME TOTAL:								
SNACK								
TIME TOTAL:								
GRAND TOTALS:								

PHYSICAL ACTIVITY

ACTIVITY	DURATION	INTENSITY	CAL/BURN

BLOOD SUGAR LOG

	BEFORE	AFTER	INSULIN

NOTES:

DAYS		DATE		WEIGHT		

SLEEP (HRS) 🌙 1 2 3 4 5 6 7 8 _____
WATER (CUP) 🥤🥤🥤🥤🥤🥤🥤🥤 ___

BREAKFAST	BEFORE	AFTER	CALORIES	CARBS (G)	ADDED SUGAR(G)	FIBER (G)	PROTEIN (G)	FAT (G)
TIME TOTAL:								
SNACK								
TIME TOTAL:								
LUNCH								
TIME TOTAL:								
SNACK								
TIME TOTAL:								

VITAMINS/MEDS/SUPPLEMENT/NOTES

DINNER	BEFORE	AFTER	CALORIES	CARBS (G)	ADDED SUGAR(G)	FIBER (G)	PROTEIN (G)	FAT (G)
TIME TOTAL:								
SNACK								
TIME TOTAL:								
GRAND TOTALS:								

PHYSICAL ACTIVITY

ACTIVITY	DURATION	INTENSITY	CAL/BURN

BLOOD SUGAR LOG

	BEFORE	AFTER	INSULIN

NOTES:

DAYS   **DATE**   **WEIGHT**

SLEEP (HRS) 1 2 3 4 5 6 7 8 ____
WATER (CUP) ⎕⎕⎕⎕⎕⎕⎕⎕ ____

BREAKFAST	BEFORE	AFTER	CALORIES	CARBS (G)	ADDED SUGAR(G)	FIBER (G)	PROTEIN (G)	FAT (G)
TIME TOTAL:								
SNACK								
TIME TOTAL:								
LUNCH								
TIME TOTAL:								
SNACK								
TIME TOTAL:								

VITAMINS/MEDS/SUPPLEMENT/NOTES

DINNER	BEFORE	AFTER	CALORIES	CARBS (G)	ADDED SUGAR(G)	FIBER (G)	PROTEIN (G)	FAT (G)
TIME TOTAL:								
SNACK								
TIME TOTAL:								
GRAND TOTALS:								

PHYSICAL ACTIVITY

ACTIVITY	DURATION	INTENSITY	CAL/BURN

BLOOD SUGAR LOG

	BEFORE	AFTER	INSULIN

NOTES:

DAYS   DATE   WEIGHT

SLEEP (HRS) 🌙 1 2 3 4 5 6 7 8 ____
WATER (CUP) ☕☕☕☕☕☕☕☕ ____

BREAKFAST	BEFORE	AFTER	CALORIES	CARBS (G)	ADDED SUGAR(G)	FIBER (G)	PROTEIN (G)	FAT (G)
TIME TOTAL:								

SNACK								
TIME TOTAL:								

LUNCH								
TIME TOTAL:								

SNACK								
TIME TOTAL:								

VITAMINS/MEDS/SUPPLEMENT/NOTES

DINNER	BEFORE	AFTER	CALORIES	CARBS (G)	ADDED SUGAR(G)	FIBER (G)	PROTEIN (G)	FAT (G)
ME	TOTAL:							
SNACK								
ME	TOTAL:							
GRAND TOTALS:								

PHYSICAL ACTIVITY

ACTIVITY	DURATION	INTENSITY	CAL/BURN

BLOOD SUGAR LOG

	BEFORE	AFTER	INSULIN

NOTES:

Made in the USA
Middletown, DE
17 November 2021

52741743R00060